Natural Probiotics Food Health Benefit

Health Benefits of Natural Probiotics

By

Casey Derry

Table of Contents

CHAPTER 1

Introduction

1.1 Definition of Natural Probiotics

Probiotics are live microorganisms that, when consumed in adequate amounts, provide health benefits to the host. The term "probiotic" is derived from the Greek words "pro," meaning "for," and "biotic," meaning "life." These microorganisms, mainly bacteria and some types of yeast, are commonly found in various foods and supplements.

Natural probiotics refer to the beneficial microorganisms that occur naturally in certain foods or are produced through fermentation processes. Unlike probiotic supplements, which are specifically formulated to contain high concentrations of specific strains, natural probiotics are present in whole foods and retain their natural composition and diversity.

These live microorganisms can have a positive impact on the human body, particularly on the gut microbiota, which refers to the trillions of microorganisms residing in our digestive system. The gut microbiota plays a crucial role in maintaining overall health and is involved in various physiological processes, including digestion, nutrient absorption, metabolism, and immune function.

The natural sources of probiotics are primarily fermented foods and beverages that have undergone a fermentation process, allowing beneficial bacteria or yeasts to multiply and thrive. Some examples of natural probiotic foods include yogurt, kefir, sauerkraut, kimchi, kombucha, tempeh, miso, and pickles, among others. These foods have a long history of consumption in different cultures and are valued not only for their taste but also for their potential health benefits.

The microorganisms present in natural probiotic foods, such as Lactobacillus and Bifidobacterium strains, have been extensively studied for their health-promoting properties. These probiotic strains have the ability to survive the harsh conditions of the digestive tract and reach the intestines, where they can exert their beneficial effects.

It is important to note that not all fermented foods contain live and active probiotics. Many commercially available products, such as pasteurized yogurt or pickles, undergo processes that kill the beneficial microorganisms. Therefore, it is crucial to look for labels indicating live and active cultures or opt for homemade or traditionally fermented foods to ensure the presence of viable probiotics.

natural probiotics refer to live microorganisms found in certain fermented foods and beverages. These probiotics have the potential to confer health benefits, particularly in relation to gut health, digestion, and immune function. Incorporating natural probiotic foods into your diet can be a delicious and nutritious way to support your overall well-being.

1.2 Importance of Probiotics for Health

Probiotics play a crucial role in maintaining and promoting health. The benefits of probiotics extend beyond just the digestive system, influencing various aspects of overall well-being. Here are some key reasons why probiotics are important for health:

1. Gut Health: Probiotics contribute to a healthy gut microbiota, which is essential for proper digestion, nutrient absorption, and gut function. They help maintain a balanced microbial community in the gut, preventing the overgrowth of harmful bacteria and supporting the growth of beneficial ones. A healthy gut microbiota is associated with

improved digestion, reduced risk of gastrointestinal disorders such as diarrhea and irritable bowel syndrome (IBS), and enhanced bowel regularity.

2. Immune Function: The gut microbiota plays a vital role in immune system development and function. Probiotics help modulate the immune response, promoting a balanced and effective immune system. They stimulate the production of certain immune cells, enhance the gut barrier function, and compete with pathogenic bacteria for resources and attachment sites. By supporting a healthy gut microbiota, probiotics can help strengthen the immune system, reducing

the risk of infections and allergies.

3. Management of Inflammatory Bowel Diseases (IBD): Inflammatory bowel diseases, such as Crohn's disease and ulcerative colitis, involve chronic inflammation of the digestive tract. Probiotics have shown promise in managing symptoms and reducing inflammation in individuals with IBD. Certain strains of probiotics have been found to decrease disease activity, improve quality of life, and reduce the need for medication in some cases.

4. Antibiotic-Associated Diarrhea and Infections: Antibiotics are known to disrupt the balance of the gut microbiota, often

leading to antibiotic-associated diarrhea and infections. Probiotics can help restore the microbial balance during and after antibiotic treatment. They help prevent the overgrowth of harmful bacteria, reduce the risk of antibiotic-associated diarrhea, and support the recovery of a healthy gut microbiota.

5. Mental Health: The gut-brain axis is a bidirectional communication system between the gut and the brain. Emerging research suggests that the gut microbiota and probiotics can influence mental health and well-being. Probiotics have been studied for their potential role in reducing symptoms of depression, anxiety, and stress.

While the exact mechanisms are still being investigated, it is believed that probiotics can modulate neurotransmitter production, reduce inflammation, and improve gut-brain signaling.

6. Skin Health: Probiotics may also have a positive impact on skin health. Imbalances in the gut microbiota can contribute to skin conditions such as acne, eczema, and rosacea. By promoting a healthy gut microbiota, probiotics may help alleviate inflammation, improve skin barrier function, and enhance the overall appearance and health of the skin.

7. Other Potential Benefits: Probiotics are a subject of ongoing research, and their

potential health benefits extend beyond the areas mentioned above. Studies suggest that probiotics may have effects on weight management, cholesterol levels, blood pressure, oral health, and vaginal health. However, further research is needed to fully understand the extent of these benefits and the specific strains and doses required.

It's important to note that the benefits of probiotics can vary depending on the specific strains and doses used. Different probiotic strains have different mechanisms of action and may exert varying effects on health. Therefore, it is recommended to consult with a healthcare professional or registered dietitian for personalized advice on incorporating probiotics into your diet or choosing appropriate probiotic supplements.

1.3 Types of Probiotics in Natural Foods

Natural foods are a rich source of various types of probiotics, each with its own unique benefits. Here are some common types of probiotics found in natural foods:

1. Lactobacillus: Lactobacillus is one of the most well-known and extensively studied genera of probiotic bacteria. It is naturally present in many fermented foods and is known for its ability to break down lactose, the sugar found in milk. Lactobacillus strains, such as Lactobacillus acidophilus, Lactobacillus

rhamnosus, and Lactobacillus casei, are commonly found in yogurt, kefir, and other fermented dairy products.

2. Bifidobacterium: Bifidobacterium is another important group of probiotic bacteria. It primarily inhabits the lower part of the digestive tract and is known to confer various health benefits. Bifidobacterium strains, including Bifidobacterium bifidum, Bifidobacterium longum, and Bifidobacterium breve, are commonly found in yogurt, kefir, and other fermented dairy products. They are also present in fermented vegetables like sauerkraut and kimchi.

3. Saccharomyces boulardii:
    Saccharomyces boulardii is a
    beneficial yeast probiotic. It is
    known for its ability to survive
    the acidic environment of the
    stomach and colonize the
    intestines. Saccharomyces
    boulardii has been extensively
    studied for its efficacy in
    managing antibiotic-associated
    diarrhea, Clostridium difficile
    infection, and other digestive
    disorders. It is often found in
    probiotic supplements and
    some fermented foods.

4. Streptococcus thermophilus:
    Streptococcus thermophilus is a
    thermophilic bacterium
    commonly used in the
    production of yogurt and other
    fermented dairy products.
    While it is not considered a

traditional probiotic due to its limited ability to survive the gastrointestinal tract, it plays a significant role in yogurt fermentation and contributes to the sensory qualities of the final product.

5. Other Probiotic Strains: Besides the aforementioned probiotic types, there are many other strains that can be found in natural foods. For instance, certain types of fermented vegetables may contain probiotic strains like Leuconostoc mesenteroides or Pediococcus pentosaceus. Fermented soy-based foods like tempeh and miso contain probiotic strains like Bacillus subtilis and Rhizopus oligosporus. Kombucha, a

fermented tea, can contain a variety of probiotic bacteria and yeasts depending on the fermentation process.

It is important to note that the specific strains and amounts of probiotics present in natural foods can vary depending on the fermentation process, ingredients, and storage conditions. Additionally, the viability and potency of probiotics in natural foods can decrease over time, so consuming them within their recommended shelf life is ideal for maximum benefit.

When choosing natural probiotic foods, it is advisable to opt for those that indicate the presence of live and active cultures on the label. This ensures that the beneficial microorganisms are still viable and can provide the intended health benefits.

As the field of probiotic research continues to evolve, new strains and types of probiotics may emerge, offering further opportunities to explore the health benefits of natural foods.

CHAPTER 2

Gut Health and Probiotics

2.1 Understanding the Gut Microbiome

The gut microbiome refers to the vast community of microorganisms, including bacteria, viruses, fungi, and other microbes, that inhabit the gastrointestinal tract. It is a complex and diverse ecosystem that plays a vital role in human health. The gut microbiome consists of trillions of microorganisms that collectively contribute to various physiological processes, including digestion, nutrient metabolism, immune function, and even mental health.

The composition of the gut microbiome is influenced by various factors, including genetics, diet, lifestyle, medications, and environmental exposures. Each person's gut microbiome is unique, with a combination of beneficial, neutral, and potentially harmful microorganisms. The balance and diversity of these microorganisms are crucial for maintaining gut health and overall well-being.

2.2 Role of Probiotics in Maintaining Gut Health

Probiotics, as beneficial microorganisms, play a significant role in maintaining gut health by influencing the composition and function of the gut microbiome. They can help restore microbial balance, enhance the growth of beneficial bacteria, and inhibit the growth of harmful microorganisms.

When consumed in adequate amounts, probiotics can:

1. Improve Gut Microbial Diversity: Probiotics contribute to a diverse and balanced gut microbiome by introducing new beneficial strains and supporting the growth of existing ones. A diverse gut microbiome is associated with better overall health and improved resilience against infections and diseases.

2. Enhance Gut Barrier Function: The gut lining acts as a barrier that prevents harmful substances from entering the bloodstream while allowing the

absorption of nutrients. Probiotics help strengthen the gut barrier by promoting the production of mucus and enhancing the tight junctions between gut cells. This barrier function is vital for preventing the translocation of harmful bacteria and toxins into the body.

3. Produce Beneficial Metabolites: Probiotics have the ability to ferment dietary fibers and other substrates, producing beneficial metabolites such as short-chain fatty acids (SCFAs). SCFAs provide an energy source for colon cells, regulate immune function, and have anti-inflammatory properties. They contribute to a healthy gut

environment and support overall gut health.

4. Modulate Immune Responses: Probiotics interact with the immune cells in the gut-associated lymphoid tissue (GALT) and help regulate immune responses. They can enhance the production of anti-inflammatory cytokines and reduce the production of pro-inflammatory cytokines, promoting a balanced immune system. This modulation of the immune response can benefit individuals with autoimmune conditions, allergies, and inflammatory bowel diseases.

5. Support Digestive Function: Probiotics aid in the digestion and absorption of nutrients by producing enzymes that break

down complex carbohydrates, proteins, and fats. They can help alleviate symptoms of digestive disorders such as lactose intolerance, diarrhea, and constipation.

2.3 Benefits of a Healthy Gut Microbiome

A healthy gut microbiome, maintained in part by probiotics, provides a range of benefits for overall health and well-being. Some of the key benefits include:

1. Improved Digestive Health: A balanced gut microbiome helps optimize digestion and nutrient absorption, reducing the risk of digestive disorders such as diarrhea, constipation, and irritable bowel syndrome (IBS).

2. Enhanced Immune Function: The gut microbiome and probiotics play a crucial role in training and modulating the immune system. A healthy gut microbiome supports a robust immune response, protecting against infections and promoting immune tolerance.

3. Management of Inflammatory Bowel Diseases (IBD): Imbalances in the gut microbiome are associated with inflammatory bowel diseases such as Crohn's disease and ulcerative colitis. Probiotics have shown promise in managing symptoms and reducing inflammation in individuals with IBD.

4. Mental Health and Well-being: The gut-brain axis is a

bidirectional communication system between the gut and the brain. A healthy gut microbiome and probiotics can influence brain function and mood regulation, potentially contributing to mental health and well-being.

5. Weight Management: The gut microbiome plays a role in energy metabolism and may influence weight regulation. Imbalances in the gut microbiome have been associated with obesity and metabolic disorders. Probiotics may help support a healthy weight by promoting a balanced gut microbiome.

6. Cardiovascular Health: Some studies suggest that a healthy gut microbiome, influenced by

probiotics, can help improve cholesterol levels and reduce the risk of cardiovascular diseases.

7. Overall Well-being: A healthy gut microbiome is linked to improved overall health, vitality, and quality of life. By supporting digestion, immune function, and other physiological processes, probiotics contribute to general well-being.

It is important to note that individual responses to probiotics may vary, and the specific benefits experienced can depend on factors such as the strains of probiotics consumed, the individual's gut microbiome composition, and overall health status. Consulting with a healthcare professional or registered dietitian can help determine the most appropriate probiotics and dosage for individual needs.

CHAPTER 3

Natural Probiotic Foods

3.1 Yogurt and Fermented Dairy Products

Yogurt and other fermented dairy products have long been recognized as excellent sources of natural probiotics. These foods undergo a fermentation process in which live cultures of beneficial bacteria convert the lactose in milk into lactic acid, giving yogurt its tangy taste and creamy texture. Here are some key points about yogurt and fermented dairy products as natural probiotics:

1. Probiotic Strains: Yogurt and fermented dairy products contain various strains of probiotic bacteria, with Lactobacillus acidophilus and Bifidobacterium bifidum being commonly found. These strains are known to survive the digestive process and reach the intestines, where they can confer health benefits.

2. Gut Health Benefits: Regular consumption of yogurt and fermented dairy products can help improve gut health by restoring and maintaining a healthy balance of beneficial bacteria in the gut. The live cultures present in these foods contribute to the diversity and

stability of the gut microbiome, supporting digestion, nutrient absorption, and overall gut function.

3. Lactose Digestion: The fermentation process in yogurt breaks down lactose, the naturally occurring sugar in milk. This makes yogurt more easily digestible for individuals with lactose intolerance or those who have difficulty digesting lactose. The beneficial bacteria in yogurt produce the enzyme lactase, which helps in the digestion of lactose.

4. Immune Support: The probiotics in yogurt and fermented dairy products can help enhance immune function. They stimulate the production

of immune cells, modulate immune responses, and promote a balanced immune system. This can lead to improved resistance against infections and a reduced risk of certain immune-related conditions.

5. Nutritional Value: In addition to probiotics, yogurt and fermented dairy products are rich sources of essential nutrients. They provide high-quality protein, calcium, vitamin D, B-vitamins, and other minerals, depending on the specific product. Choosing low-fat or non-fat varieties can also help support a healthy diet.

6. Product Varieties: Yogurt comes in various forms and flavors to suit different

preferences. From plain yogurt to fruit-flavored options, Greek yogurt, skyr, and kefir, there are numerous choices available. However, it is important to note that not all commercially available yogurts contain live and active cultures. Look for labels that specifically mention the presence of probiotics or live cultures to ensure you are getting the maximum benefits.

7. Homemade Fermentation: Making yogurt at home is also an option for those who prefer a DIY approach. Homemade yogurt allows you to have control over the ingredients and the fermentation process. By using a starter culture containing live and active

probiotic strains, you can create your own probiotic-rich yogurt.

When selecting yogurt or fermented dairy products as probiotic sources, it is advisable to choose those with minimal added sugars and artificial additives. Plain yogurt or those sweetened with natural sweeteners like honey or fruit can be healthier options.

It is worth noting that individuals with dairy allergies or lactose intolerance may need to explore non-dairy alternatives such as coconut milk or almond milk-based yogurts. These products can also provide probiotics, although the strains and concentrations may vary compared to traditional dairy-based options.

Overall, incorporating yogurt and other fermented dairy products into your diet can be a delicious way to obtain natural probiotics and support gut health.

3.2 Kefir

Kefir is a fermented dairy product that has gained popularity as a natural probiotic food. It is made by adding kefir grains, a combination of bacteria and yeasts, to milk and allowing them to ferment. Here are some key points about kefir as a natural probiotic:

1. Probiotic Strains: Kefir contains a diverse range of probiotic bacteria and yeasts. The exact composition of kefir grains can vary, but common probiotic strains found in kefir include Lactobacillus species (such as Lactobacillus acidophilus, Lactobacillus

kefiri) and Bifidobacterium
species (such as
Bifidobacterium bifidum). The
yeasts Saccharomyces
cerevisiae and Kluyveromyces
marxianus are also commonly
present.

2. Probiotic Benefits: Kefir is
    known for its potential to
    promote gut health. The live
    cultures in kefir can help
    restore and maintain a healthy
    balance of bacteria in the gut
    microbiome, which supports
    digestion, nutrient absorption,
    and immune function. The
    diverse probiotic strains in kefir
    can have different mechanisms
    of action and may offer
    additional health benefits
    beyond those provided by
    individual strains.

3. Lactose Digestion: Like yogurt, kefir is fermented, which breaks down lactose, making it easier to digest for individuals with lactose intolerance. The beneficial bacteria in kefir produce lactase, the enzyme needed to break down lactose. Therefore, kefir can be a suitable option for those who are lactose intolerant but can tolerate small amounts of lactose.

4. Nutritional Value: Kefir is not only a source of probiotics but also a nutrient-dense food. It is rich in high-quality protein, calcium, vitamin D, B-vitamins, and minerals. Kefir made from whole milk is higher in fat, while kefir made from low-fat or non-fat milk

options can be lower in calories and fat content.

5. Versatility and Consumption: Kefir has a tangy and slightly effervescent taste, and its texture is often described as drinkable yogurt. It can be enjoyed on its own or used in various recipes, such as smoothies, salad dressings, or as a substitute for buttermilk in baking. It is recommended to start with small amounts of kefir and gradually increase intake to allow the body to adjust to the probiotics.

6. Homemade Kefir: Kefir can be made at home using kefir grains and milk. The grains are reusable, and the fermentation process typically takes around 24-48 hours. Making kefir at

home allows you to have control over the quality of ingredients and the fermentation time. However, it is important to handle kefir grains with care and follow proper hygiene practices to prevent contamination.

7. Non-Dairy Kefir: While traditional kefir is made with dairy milk, non-dairy alternatives such as coconut milk, almond milk, or soy milk can also be used to make non-dairy kefir. Non-dairy kefir provides options for individuals who are lactose intolerant or have dairy allergies but still want to enjoy the benefits of probiotics.

As with any probiotic food, it's important to be mindful of personal tolerance and preferences. Some individuals may experience temporary digestive discomfort when first introducing kefir into their diet due to the changes in gut microbiota. It is recommended to start with small amounts and gradually increase intake.

kefir is a fermented dairy product containing a diverse range of probiotic bacteria and yeasts. It offers potential benefits for gut health, lactose digestion, and nutrient intake. Whether made at home or purchased commercially, kefir can be a valuable addition to a balanced diet for those seeking natural probiotics.

3.3 Sauerkraut and Fermented Vegetables

Sauerkraut and other fermented vegetables are popular natural probiotic foods that provide a host of health benefits. Fermented vegetables undergo a process called lacto-fermentation, in which beneficial bacteria convert the sugars in the vegetables into lactic acid. Sauerkraut, made from fermented cabbage, is a well-known example. Here are key points about sauerkraut and fermented vegetables as natural probiotics:

1. Probiotic Strains: Sauerkraut and fermented vegetables contain a range of beneficial bacteria, primarily from the Lactobacillus genus. Lactic acid bacteria, including Lactobacillus plantarum,

Lactobacillus brevis, and Lactobacillus fermentum, are commonly found in these fermented foods. These strains can survive the acidic environment of the stomach and provide health benefits when consumed.

2. Gut Health Benefits: Sauerkraut and fermented vegetables support gut health by introducing beneficial bacteria to the gut microbiome. The live cultures in these foods contribute to a diverse microbial community in the gut, aiding digestion, promoting nutrient absorption, and maintaining a balanced gut microbiota. The presence of probiotics in sauerkraut can

also help alleviate digestive issues such as bloating and gas.

3. Nutritional Value: Fermented vegetables, including sauerkraut, retain many of the nutrients present in their raw form, such as fiber, vitamins (C, K, and B-vitamins), and minerals (iron, potassium). Fermentation can increase the bioavailability of certain nutrients, making them more easily absorbed by the body. Additionally, sauerkraut is low in calories and fat.

4. Antioxidant and Anti-inflammatory Properties: The fermentation process enhances the antioxidant content of sauerkraut and fermented vegetables. Antioxidants help protect the body against

oxidative stress and inflammation, which are linked to various chronic diseases. The lactic acid bacteria in sauerkraut produce compounds that possess anti-inflammatory properties, further contributing to overall health.

5. Digestive Enzymes: Fermented vegetables contain natural digestive enzymes that can aid in the breakdown and absorption of nutrients. These enzymes can enhance digestion, particularly for individuals with compromised digestive function.

6. Versatility and Consumption: Sauerkraut and fermented vegetables can be enjoyed as condiments, added to salads, sandwiches, or used in various

recipes. They add a tangy and flavorful element to dishes, enhancing taste and texture. It is recommended to consume them in moderation due to their high salt content. Opting for homemade or traditionally fermented varieties without added preservatives or excessive salt is preferred.

7. Homemade Fermentation: Making sauerkraut and fermented vegetables at home is a popular option for those interested in the art of fermentation. It allows for customization of flavors and provides control over the fermentation process. Basic ingredients typically include vegetables, salt, and water, and the fermentation period can

range from several days to weeks.

It's important to note that commercial varieties of sauerkraut and fermented vegetables may undergo pasteurization or undergo processes that kill the beneficial bacteria. Therefore, it is important to choose products that specifically state "live and active cultures" or opt for homemade versions to ensure the presence of viable probiotics.

sauerkraut and fermented vegetables are natural probiotic foods that offer numerous health benefits. They support gut health, provide valuable nutrients, and contribute to overall well-being. Including these probiotic-rich foods as part of a balanced diet can be a delicious and healthy way to enhance gut health.

3.4 Kimchi

Kimchi is a traditional Korean fermented vegetable dish that has gained popularity worldwide for its unique flavors and health benefits. It is typically made from cabbage, radishes, and various seasonings. Here are key points about kimchi as a natural probiotic food:

1. Probiotic Strains: Kimchi contains a diverse range of beneficial bacteria, mainly from the lactic acid bacteria family. Lactobacillus plantarum, Lactobacillus brevis, and Leuconostoc species are commonly found in kimchi. These probiotic strains contribute to the fermentation process and provide health benefits when consumed.

2. Gut Health Benefits: Kimchi is known for its positive effects on gut health. The live cultures in kimchi help restore and maintain a healthy balance of bacteria in the gut microbiome. The probiotics in kimchi can enhance digestion, promote nutrient absorption, and support a balanced gut microbiota. Regular consumption of kimchi has been associated with improved gut function and reduced risk of digestive disorders.

3. Nutritional Value: Kimchi is rich in vitamins (such as vitamin C, vitamin K, and various B-vitamins), minerals (calcium, iron, and potassium), dietary fiber, and antioxidants. Fermentation enhances the

bioavailability of these nutrients, making them more easily absorbed by the body. Kimchi is typically low in calories and fat, making it a nutritious addition to a balanced diet.

4. Antioxidant and Anti-inflammatory Properties: Kimchi contains antioxidants and bioactive compounds that possess anti-inflammatory properties. These compounds help protect against oxidative stress and inflammation, which are associated with chronic diseases. The fermentation process increases the antioxidant content of kimchi, further enhancing its health benefits.

5. Immune Support: The probiotics and bioactive compounds in kimchi can help support immune function. Probiotics play a role in regulating immune responses, while the compounds in kimchi can enhance immune cell activity and strengthen the immune system. Regular consumption of kimchi may contribute to better immune health and reduced susceptibility to infections.

6. Flavor and Culinary Uses: Kimchi is known for its distinct and vibrant flavors, ranging from spicy and tangy to savory and slightly sour. It is a versatile ingredient that can be enjoyed on its own as a side dish, incorporated into main

dishes like stir-fries and stews, or used as a flavoring agent in various recipes. Kimchi adds depth and complexity to dishes, enhancing taste and providing a unique culinary experience.

7. Store-Bought vs. Homemade: Kimchi is available in most grocery stores, but it's important to note that commercial varieties may undergo processes, such as pasteurization or extended shelf-life treatments, which can affect the presence of live probiotics. Homemade kimchi allows for more control over the fermentation process and ensures the preservation of the beneficial bacteria. Making kimchi at home also allows for

customization of flavors and ingredients.

When consuming kimchi, it is important to be mindful of its salt content, as some varieties can be high in sodium. Individuals on sodium-restricted diets should consider consuming kimchi in moderation or opt for lower-sodium versions.

kimchi is a natural probiotic food with numerous health benefits. It supports gut health, provides essential nutrients, and contributes to overall well-being. Adding kimchi to your diet can introduce unique flavors and promote a diverse gut microbiome.

3.5 Kombucha

Kombucha is a fermented tea beverage that has gained popularity as a natural probiotic drink. It is made by fermenting sweetened tea with a symbiotic culture of bacteria and yeast (SCOBY). Here are key points about kombucha as a natural probiotic:

1. Probiotic Strains: Kombucha contains a variety of beneficial bacteria and yeasts. Common probiotic strains found in kombucha include species from the Lactobacillus, Acetobacter, and Saccharomyces genera. The specific strains can vary depending on the fermentation process and the starter culture used.

2. Gut Health Benefits: Kombucha can support gut health by introducing live cultures of beneficial bacteria to the gut microbiome. These

probiotics help maintain a diverse and balanced microbial community in the gut, promoting digestion, nutrient absorption, and overall gut function. Regular consumption of kombucha has been associated with improved gut health and digestive well-being.

3. Antioxidant Properties: Kombucha is rich in antioxidants, including polyphenols, which are beneficial compounds that help protect against oxidative stress and inflammation. The fermentation process increases the antioxidant content of kombucha, making it a potential source of health-promoting compounds.

4. Potential Detoxifying Effects:
   Some proponents claim that
   kombucha has detoxifying
   effects due to its ability to
   support liver function.
   However, scientific evidence
   on this specific claim is limited,
   and more research is needed to
   establish the extent and
   mechanisms of any potential
   detoxification effects.

5. Probiotic Diversity: Kombucha
   can provide a wide range of
   probiotic strains, contributing
   to a diverse gut microbiome.
   The presence of different
   strains in kombucha may offer
   additional health benefits
   beyond those provided by
   individual strains, potentially
   supporting immune function
   and overall well-being.

6. Carbonation and Taste: Kombucha is naturally carbonated, giving it a slightly effervescent quality. It has a tangy and slightly acidic taste, which can vary depending on the fermentation process and added flavors. Kombucha is available in a variety of flavors, including fruit-infused variations.

7. Store-Bought vs. Homemade: Kombucha is readily available in many grocery stores, often in bottled form. However, it is essential to choose products that are unpasteurized and contain live cultures to ensure the presence of viable probiotics. Homemade kombucha allows for more control over the ingredients and

fermentation process. However,
it is important to follow proper
brewing procedures to prevent
contamination and ensure a safe
and healthy final product.

It is worth noting that kombucha is
typically made with black or green
tea, which naturally contains caffeine.
However, the fermentation process
can reduce the caffeine content.
Nevertheless, individuals who are
sensitive to caffeine should be
mindful of their kombucha
consumption.

While kombucha is generally
considered safe for most individuals,
it may not be suitable for everyone.
Individuals with compromised
immune systems, pregnant or
breastfeeding women, and those with
certain health conditions should

consult with a healthcare professional before consuming kombucha.

kombucha is a natural probiotic beverage with potential health benefits. It supports gut health, provides antioxidants, and offers a unique taste experience. Incorporating kombucha into your diet can be a refreshing way to introduce beneficial probiotics.

3.6 Tempeh and Miso

Tempeh and miso are fermented soy-based products that serve as natural probiotics. They are widely consumed in Asian cuisines and offer various health benefits. Here are key points about tempeh and miso as natural probiotic foods:

1. Probiotic Strains: Tempeh and miso contain beneficial bacteria and yeasts that contribute to the fermentation process. The specific strains vary depending on the fermentation conditions and starter cultures used. Some common probiotic strains found in tempeh and miso include species from the Bacillus, Aspergillus, and Rhizopus genera.

2. Gut Health Benefits: The live cultures present in tempeh and miso can support gut health by introducing beneficial microorganisms to the gut microbiome. These probiotics help maintain a balanced gut microbial community, promoting digestion, nutrient absorption, and overall gut

function. Regular consumption of tempeh and miso has been associated with improved gut health and digestive well-being.

3. Nutritional Value: Tempeh and miso are highly nutritious. They are rich sources of plant-based protein, essential amino acids, fiber, vitamins (such as B-vitamins and vitamin K), and minerals (including iron, calcium, and magnesium). Fermentation can enhance the bioavailability and digestibility of these nutrients, making them more accessible to the body.

4. Soy Benefits: Tempeh and miso are derived from soybeans, which offer additional health benefits. Soybeans are rich in isoflavones, phytoestrogens that have been associated with

various health effects, including potential protective effects against certain chronic diseases such as cardiovascular disease and certain types of cancer.

5. Versatility and Culinary Uses: Tempeh and miso can be used in a variety of culinary applications. Tempeh has a firm, nutty texture and can be sliced, marinated, grilled, or used as a meat substitute in various dishes. Miso is a fermented paste that adds depth of flavor to soups, stews, marinades, dressings, and sauces. Both tempeh and miso offer unique flavors that can enhance a wide range of recipes.

6. Fermentation Process: Tempeh is made by fermenting cooked

soybeans with a starter culture, usually a type of fungus called Rhizopus oligosporus. The fermentation process binds the soybeans together, forming a solid cake with a distinct texture and flavor. Miso, on the other hand, is made by fermenting soybeans, along with salt and a mold culture called Aspergillus oryzae, which breaks down the soybeans into a paste.

7. Gluten-Free and Dairy-Free Options: Tempeh and miso are naturally gluten-free and dairy-free, making them suitable for individuals with gluten sensitivity, celiac disease, or lactose intolerance. They offer plant-based alternatives for individuals looking to

incorporate probiotics into their diet without consuming animal products.

When purchasing tempeh and miso, it is important to choose products that are minimally processed and preferably made with organic, non-genetically modified soybeans. Some commercial varieties may contain added ingredients or preservatives, so reading labels and choosing products with simple ingredient lists is recommended.

Tempeh and miso are natural probiotic foods derived from fermented soybeans. They offer health benefits such as supporting gut health, providing essential nutrients, and adding unique flavors to dishes. Incorporating tempeh and miso into your diet can be a delicious and nutritious way to enjoy the benefits of natural probiotics.

3.7 Pickles

Pickles are a popular fermented food enjoyed worldwide. They are made by immersing cucumbers or other vegetables in a brine solution or vinegar and allowing them to ferment. Here are key points about pickles as a natural probiotic food:

1. Probiotic Potential: While not all pickles are made through fermentation, those that are fermented offer probiotic benefits. Fermented pickles undergo a natural fermentation process, where beneficial bacteria convert the sugars present in the vegetables into lactic acid, creating a sour and

tangy flavor. This fermentation process introduces live cultures of beneficial bacteria to the pickles.

2. Probiotic Strains: The probiotic strains in fermented pickles can vary, as they are dependent on the specific bacteria present during the fermentation process. Lactic acid bacteria, such as Lactobacillus species and Pediococcus species, are commonly found in fermented pickles. These strains can survive the digestive process and provide potential health benefits.

3. Gut Health Benefits: Fermented pickles can contribute to gut health by introducing beneficial bacteria to the gut microbiome. The live cultures present in

these pickles help support a diverse and balanced gut microbial community, aiding digestion, nutrient absorption, and overall gut function. Regular consumption of fermented pickles has been associated with improved gut health and digestive well-being.

4. Nutritional Value: Pickles, both fermented and non-fermented, can be a source of vitamins, minerals, and fiber. Fermented pickles also retain the nutrients present in the vegetables used, such as cucumbers, radishes, or carrots. However, it's worth noting that pickles made with vinegar alone, without fermentation, may not offer the same probiotic benefits as fermented pickles.

5. Sodium Content: Pickles, particularly commercially available varieties, can be high in sodium due to the brine solution used for pickling. Individuals on sodium-restricted diets should be mindful of their pickle consumption and opt for lower sodium varieties or homemade pickles with reduced salt content.

6. Versatility and Culinary Uses: Pickles can be enjoyed as a condiment, added to sandwiches, salads, or eaten on their own as a snack. They provide a tangy and refreshing flavor that complements various dishes. The versatility of pickles allows for creative

culinary applications and adds a satisfying crunch to meals.

7. Homemade Pickles: Making pickles at home allows for control over the fermentation process and ingredients used. Homemade fermented pickles can be made with a variety of vegetables and flavorings, allowing for customization and experimentation with different flavors and textures.

It's important to note that not all pickles found in stores undergo fermentation. Many commercially available pickles are made through quick pickling methods using vinegar or other acidic solutions, which do not provide the same probiotic benefits as fermented pickles. Reading labels and looking for phrases like "fermented" or "naturally fermented" can help identify probiotic-rich pickles.

fermented pickles offer probiotic benefits and can support gut health. They provide a tangy flavor, crunch, and can be enjoyed as a condiment or snack. Incorporating fermented pickles into your diet can be a tasty way to introduce beneficial bacteria to your gut microbiome.

3.8 Traditional Buttermilk

Traditional buttermilk is a fermented dairy product that is different from the cultured buttermilk commonly found in stores today. It is a byproduct of churning butter from cream. Here are key points about traditional buttermilk as a natural probiotic food:

1. Fermentation Process:
    Traditional buttermilk is made
    by collecting the liquid left
    after butter is churned from
    cream. The cream is allowed to
    naturally ferment, usually
    overnight, at room temperature.
    During fermentation, beneficial
    bacteria convert lactose into
    lactic acid, giving buttermilk its
    tangy flavor.

2. Probiotic Strains: The
    fermentation of traditional
    buttermilk introduces various
    probiotic bacteria to the drink.
    These bacteria typically include
    species from the Lactobacillus
    and Streptococcus genera, such
    as Lactobacillus acidophilus
    and Lactobacillus delbrueckii
    subsp. bulgaricus. These strains
    contribute to the probiotic

properties of traditional buttermilk.

3. Gut Health Benefits: Traditional buttermilk supports gut health by introducing beneficial bacteria to the gut microbiome. The live cultures in buttermilk help promote a diverse and balanced gut microbial community, aiding digestion, nutrient absorption, and overall gut function. Regular consumption of traditional buttermilk can contribute to improved gut health and digestive well-being.

4. Nutritional Value: Traditional buttermilk retains many of the nutrients present in the cream used to make butter. It is a good source of protein, calcium, phosphorus, vitamin B12, and

other vitamins and minerals.
However, traditional buttermilk
may have a higher fat content
than cultured buttermilk or low-
fat milk.

5. Culinary Uses: Traditional
    buttermilk is used in various
    culinary applications. It can be
    enjoyed as a refreshing
    beverage on its own or used as
    an ingredient in baking,
    marinades, salad dressings, and
    other recipes. Traditional
    buttermilk adds a tangy flavor
    and helps tenderize and moisten
    baked goods.

It's important to note that the
buttermilk commonly available in
stores today is often cultured
buttermilk, which is made by
introducing specific bacteria to
pasteurized milk. While cultured

buttermilk also contains beneficial bacteria, it may have a different composition and flavor compared to traditional buttermilk.

3.9 Other Natural Probiotic Foods

In addition to the specific foods mentioned above, there are various other natural probiotic foods that offer health benefits. Here are some examples:

1. Apple Cider Vinegar (with the "mother"): Unfiltered apple cider vinegar containing the "mother" is a fermented product that can contain beneficial bacteria. It is believed to have potential digestive benefits when consumed in moderation.

2. Sourdough Bread: True sourdough bread is made through a natural fermentation process using a sourdough starter, which contains wild yeast and lactic acid bacteria. This fermentation process contributes to a tangy flavor and can increase the digestibility and nutritional value of the bread.

3. Natto: Natto is a traditional Japanese food made from fermented soybeans. It contains a specific probiotic strain called Bacillus subtilis, which has been associated with potential cardiovascular and bone health benefits.

4. Kvass: Kvass is a fermented beverage traditionally made from rye bread or other grains.

It contains lactobacilli and other beneficial bacteria and is known for its probiotic properties. Kvass can also be made from beets or other vegetables.

5. Raw Cheese: Some varieties of raw, unpasteurized cheese contain live cultures of beneficial bacteria. These cheeses undergo natural fermentation and can offer probiotic benefits. However, it's important to ensure the safety and quality of raw cheeses by sourcing them from reputable sources.

6. Fermented Soy Products: Besides tempeh and miso, other fermented soy products like soy sauce, soybean paste (doenjang), and fermented soy

milk (such as shoyu and tamari) can contain probiotic bacteria and provide health benefits.

When incorporating natural probiotic foods into your diet, it's important to consider personal preferences, dietary restrictions, and any potential allergies or intolerances. It's recommended to introduce these foods gradually and listen to your body's response. Consulting with a healthcare professional or registered dietitian can provide personalized guidance on incorporating probiotics into your diet.

CHAPTER 4

Health Benefits of Natural Probiotics

4.1 Improved Digestive Health

One of the primary health benefits associated with natural probiotics is their ability to improve digestive health. Probiotics help maintain a healthy balance of bacteria in the gut microbiome, which is crucial for optimal digestion and nutrient absorption. Here are some specific ways natural probiotics can support digestive health:

a) Restoring Gut Microbiome Balance: The gut is home to trillions of bacteria, both beneficial and potentially harmful. When the balance of these bacteria is disrupted, it can lead to digestive issues such as bloating, gas, diarrhea, or constipation. Natural probiotics help restore this balance by increasing the population of beneficial bacteria in the gut, improving overall digestive function.

b) Enhancing Nutrient Absorption: The presence of a diverse and balanced gut microbiome is essential for proper nutrient absorption. Probiotics can help break down food and release nutrients, making them more accessible to the body. For example, certain probiotic strains produce enzymes that assist in the digestion of lactose, aiding individuals with lactose intolerance.

c) Alleviating Digestive Disorders:
Research suggests that natural
probiotics can provide relief for
certain digestive disorders. Conditions
such as irritable bowel syndrome
(IBS), inflammatory bowel disease
(IBD), and antibiotic-associated
diarrhea have shown potential
improvement with the use of
probiotics. Probiotics may help reduce
inflammation, restore gut barrier
function, and alleviate symptoms
associated with these conditions.

d) Preventing and Treating Diarrhea:
Probiotics, particularly strains like
Lactobacillus rhamnosus and
Saccharomyces boulardii, have been
shown to be effective in preventing
and treating various types of diarrhea.
They can help restore the balance of
gut bacteria disrupted by infections,
antibiotics, or other factors, thereby

reducing the severity and duration of diarrhea.

4.2 Enhanced Immune Function

Another significant health benefit of natural probiotics is their ability to enhance immune function. The gut microbiome plays a vital role in immune system regulation, and maintaining a healthy balance of gut bacteria can support a robust immune response. Here's how natural probiotics contribute to improved immune function:

a) Immune System Stimulation: Natural probiotics interact with the immune cells in the gut-associated lymphoid tissue, stimulating the production of immune cells and promoting a balanced immune response. They can help modulate the immune system, enhancing its ability to fight off infections and respond to pathogens effectively.

b) Protection Against Pathogens: Probiotics can compete with and inhibit the growth of harmful bacteria, preventing their colonization in the gut. By creating an environment that is unfavorable for pathogenic bacteria, probiotics help protect against infections and reduce the risk of gastrointestinal illnesses.

c) Reduction of Allergies and Autoimmune Reactions: Emerging research suggests that the gut microbiome has an impact on the development and regulation of allergies and autoimmune conditions. Natural probiotics may help regulate immune responses, reducing the risk or severity of allergic reactions and mitigating autoimmune reactions.

d) Maintenance of Intestinal Barrier Function: A healthy gut barrier is essential for immune health. Probiotics can help strengthen the integrity of the intestinal lining, preventing the translocation of harmful substances from the gut into the bloodstream. This can reduce the risk of systemic inflammation and support overall immune function.

It's important to note that while natural probiotics can contribute to improved digestive health and enhanced immune function, their specific effects may vary depending on the individual, the probiotic strains used, and the underlying health conditions. Consulting with a healthcare professional is advisable, especially for individuals with specific health concerns or conditions.

4.3 Management of Inflammatory Bowel Diseases

Inflammatory bowel diseases (IBD), including Crohn's disease and ulcerative colitis, are chronic conditions characterized by inflammation in the digestive tract. Natural probiotics have shown promise in managing and reducing symptoms associated with these conditions. Here's how probiotics can contribute to the management of inflammatory bowel diseases:

a) Reduction of Inflammation: Probiotics can help modulate the inflammatory response in the gut by promoting a balanced immune system and reducing the production of pro-inflammatory compounds. This can help alleviate inflammation and provide relief from symptoms such as abdominal pain, diarrhea, and bowel irregularities.

b) Maintenance of Gut Barrier Function: The integrity of the gut barrier is compromised in individuals with inflammatory bowel diseases. Probiotics can help strengthen the gut barrier, preventing the translocation of harmful substances and pathogens from the gut into the bloodstream. By improving gut barrier function, probiotics may help reduce inflammation and prevent flare-ups of IBD.

c) Restoration of Gut Microbiome Balance: Imbalances in the gut microbiome are associated with inflammatory bowel diseases. Probiotics contribute to the restoration of a diverse and balanced gut microbial community, promoting a healthier gut environment. This can help alleviate symptoms and support overall gut health in individuals with IBD.

d) Reduction of Disease Flares: Some studies suggest that certain probiotic strains, such as certain strains of Lactobacillus and Bifidobacterium, may help reduce the frequency and severity of disease flares in individuals with inflammatory bowel diseases. Probiotics may help maintain disease remission and provide long-term management support.

It's important to note that while probiotics can offer benefits for individuals with inflammatory bowel diseases, the effectiveness may vary among individuals, and not all strains may be equally effective. Consulting with a healthcare professional and working with a gastroenterologist or registered dietitian experienced in IBD management is crucial for personalized advice and recommendations.

4.4 Potential Weight Management Effects

There is some evidence to suggest that natural probiotics may have a potential role in weight management. While weight management is complex and multifactorial, here are some ways probiotics might influence weight:

a) Regulation of Appetite and Satiety: Probiotics can influence the production and release of certain hormones involved in appetite regulation, such as ghrelin and leptin. By modulating these hormones, probiotics may help promote feelings of fullness and reduce overall calorie intake, potentially supporting weight management efforts.

b) Modulation of Gut Microbiota Composition: The gut microbiome composition has been linked to weight and metabolism. Certain probiotic strains may help maintain a diverse and balanced gut microbiota associated with a healthier body weight. Studies have shown that individuals with a more diverse gut microbiome tend to have a lower risk of obesity.

c) Metabolism of Dietary Components: Some probiotic strains have been found to influence the metabolism of dietary components, such as fiber and fats. For example, certain strains can break down dietary fibers into short-chain fatty acids, which may have benefits for metabolism and weight management.

d) Reduction of Systemic Inflammation: Chronic low-grade inflammation is associated with obesity and metabolic disorders. Probiotics may help reduce systemic inflammation by improving gut health, supporting a healthy gut barrier, and modulating immune responses. By reducing inflammation, probiotics may indirectly contribute to weight management.

While research suggests a potential role for probiotics in weight management, it's important to note that individual responses can vary, and probiotics alone are not a magic solution for weight loss. Lifestyle factors, including diet and physical activity, play a significant role in weight management. Incorporating probiotics as part of a balanced diet and healthy lifestyle is recommended for overall well-being.

As always, consulting with a healthcare professional or registered dietitian can provide personalized guidance on incorporating probiotics into a weight management plan.

4.5 Mental Health and Probiotics

Emerging research suggests a potential link between gut health and mental health, indicating that natural probiotics may have a positive impact on mental well-being. While more studies are needed, here are some ways probiotics might influence mental health:

a) Gut-Brain Axis: The gut and the brain are interconnected through the gut-brain axis, which involves bidirectional communication between the central nervous system and the gut microbiota. The gut microbiota can influence neurotransmitter production, immune function, and neuroinflammation, all of which are implicated in mental health conditions.

b) Serotonin Production: Probiotics may play a role in the production and regulation of serotonin, a neurotransmitter that plays a key role in mood regulation. Serotonin is predominantly produced in the gut, and a healthy gut microbiota composition is essential for its synthesis. Some probiotic strains may enhance serotonin production, potentially influencing mood and mental well-being.

c) Stress Response and Anxiety: Probiotics have been shown to modulate the body's stress response and reduce anxiety-like behaviors in animal studies. They may help regulate the hypothalamic-pituitary-adrenal (HPA) axis, which is involved in the stress response. By promoting a balanced stress response, probiotics may contribute to improved mental health.

d) Immune System and Inflammation: The gut microbiota composition can influence immune function and systemic inflammation, both of which are implicated in mental health conditions. Probiotics may help regulate immune responses and reduce inflammation, potentially impacting mental well-being.

While the research is promising, it's important to note that the effects of probiotics on mental health are still being studied, and individual responses may vary. Mental health conditions are complex, and probiotics should not be considered a standalone treatment. It is crucial to seek professional advice from a healthcare provider or mental health professional for a comprehensive approach to mental health management.

4.6 Skin Health and Probiotics

There is growing interest in the relationship between gut health and skin health, and some studies suggest that natural probiotics can potentially benefit certain skin conditions. Here are some ways probiotics might influence skin health:

a) Modulation of Skin Microbiome: The skin has its own microbiome, and imbalances in the skin microbiota can contribute to skin conditions such as acne, eczema, and rosacea. Probiotics may help maintain a healthy balance of beneficial bacteria on the skin, promoting a favorable environment for skin health.

b) Reduction of Inflammation: Probiotics have been found to have anti-inflammatory effects, both systemically and locally. By reducing systemic inflammation and modulating immune responses, probiotics may help alleviate inflammation-related skin conditions and promote healthier skin.

c) Strengthening Skin Barrier: A healthy skin barrier is crucial for maintaining skin health and preventing moisture loss. Some probiotic strains have been shown to enhance the production of ceramides, which are important components of the skin barrier. By strengthening the skin barrier, probiotics may help improve skin hydration and protect against external irritants.

d) Potential Role in Acne Management: Preliminary studies suggest that certain probiotic strains may have a positive impact on acne management. Probiotics may help reduce inflammation, inhibit the growth of acne-causing bacteria, and regulate sebum production, which can contribute to improved acne symptoms.

While probiotics show promise for skin health, it's important to note that research is ongoing, and individual responses may vary. It's recommended to consult with a dermatologist or healthcare professional for personalized advice on incorporating probiotics into a skincare routine or addressing specific skin concerns.

As with any health-related concerns, it's important to adopt a holistic approach, considering lifestyle factors, skincare practices, and seeking professional guidance when needed. Probiotics should be seen as a complementary strategy rather than a standalone solution for skin health.

4.7 Other Potential Health Benefits

In addition to the specific health benefits mentioned above, natural probiotics may have potential benefits in other areas of health. While more research is needed to fully understand their effects, here are some other potential health benefits associated with probiotics:

a) Heart Health: Some studies suggest that certain probiotic strains may have a positive impact on heart health. Probiotics may help lower blood pressure, reduce LDL cholesterol levels, and improve markers of cardiovascular health. However, more research is needed to establish the specific strains and dosages that are most effective.

b) Oral Health: The oral cavity is home to its own microbial community, and imbalances in oral bacteria can contribute to dental issues such as tooth decay and gum disease. Some probiotic strains, when administered orally or through specific dental products, may help maintain oral health by promoting a balanced oral microbiota and reducing the risk of dental problems.

c) Allergies and Asthma: Emerging research suggests a potential link between gut health, the immune system, and allergic conditions such as allergies and asthma. Probiotics may help regulate immune responses and modulate allergic reactions, potentially reducing the severity of symptoms in individuals with these conditions. However, more studies are needed to establish specific strains and their effectiveness.

d) Women's Health: Certain probiotic strains may offer benefits for women's health. For example, specific strains have shown promise in preventing and managing vaginal infections such as bacterial vaginosis and yeast infections. Additionally, probiotics may contribute to urinary tract health and support a balanced vaginal microbiome.

e) Metabolic Health: Probiotics may have potential effects on metabolic health, including glucose metabolism, insulin sensitivity, and lipid profile. Some studies suggest that certain probiotic strains may help improve markers associated with metabolic disorders such as type 2 diabetes and obesity. However, more research is needed to fully understand their impact and identify the most effective strains and dosages.

It's important to note that while probiotics show promise in these areas, the specific strains, dosages, and formulations that offer the most benefits are still being investigated. Additionally, individual responses to probiotics may vary, and their effectiveness can depend on factors such as the individual's health status, the specific condition being addressed, and other lifestyle factors.

Consulting with a healthcare professional or registered dietitian is advisable for personalized advice on incorporating probiotics into your health routine and addressing specific health concerns. They can provide guidance on selecting appropriate probiotic products and help determine the best approach for your individual needs.

CHAPTER 5

Incorporating Natural Probiotics into Your Diet

5.1 Choosing the Right Probiotic Foods

When incorporating natural probiotics into your diet, it's important to choose the right foods that contain live cultures of beneficial bacteria. Here are some tips for selecting probiotic-rich foods:

a) Look for Fermented Foods: Fermented foods are a good source of natural probiotics. Look for foods that have undergone a fermentation process, such as yogurt, kefir, sauerkraut, kimchi, tempeh, miso, and pickles. Check the labels or ingredient lists to ensure that the product contains live cultures or is labeled as fermented.

b) Check for Live Cultures: Not all fermented foods contain live cultures of beneficial bacteria. Some commercially available products, especially those that have been pasteurized or undergo extended shelf-life treatments, may not have live probiotic cultures. Look for labels that specify the presence of live or active cultures to ensure you're getting the probiotic benefits.

c) Opt for Unpasteurized Varieties: Pasteurization is a heat treatment process that kills bacteria, including beneficial probiotics. Choose unpasteurized or raw versions of fermented foods when available, as they are more likely to contain live cultures. However, it's important to handle and store unpasteurized foods properly to ensure safety.

d) Consider Diversity of Strains: Aim for a diverse range of probiotic strains in your diet. Different strains offer unique health benefits, so incorporating a variety of fermented foods can help promote a more diverse gut microbiome. Experiment with different probiotic-rich foods to introduce a wider range of beneficial bacteria into your system.

e) Personal Preferences and Dietary Needs: Choose probiotic foods that align with your personal preferences and dietary needs. For example, if you're lactose intolerant or have dairy restrictions, consider non-dairy options like plant-based yogurts, kefir made from non-dairy milk, or fermented vegetables. Find probiotic foods that you enjoy and can easily incorporate into your daily routine.

5.2 Tips for Fermenting Foods at Home

If you're interested in fermenting foods at home to create your own probiotic-rich options, here are some tips to get started:

a) Start with Simple Fermented Foods: Begin with simple fermentation projects that are beginner-friendly and require minimal equipment. Sauerkraut, pickles, or kombucha are good options for beginners. As you gain confidence and experience, you can explore more complex ferments like kimchi or homemade yogurt.

b) Use High-Quality Ingredients: Choose fresh, high-quality ingredients for fermentation. Select organic fruits, vegetables, or dairy (if making fermented dairy products). The quality of the ingredients can affect the taste, texture, and overall outcome of the fermentation process.

c) Follow Proper Sanitation: Cleanliness is essential during fermentation to avoid contamination by harmful bacteria. Ensure that all utensils, containers, and equipment are properly cleaned and sanitized before use. Proper sanitation helps create a favorable environment for the growth of beneficial bacteria.

d) Follow Recipes and Guidelines: Follow reliable recipes or guidelines when fermenting foods at home. These resources will provide instructions on ingredient ratios, fermentation times, and storage conditions. It's important to follow the recommended guidelines to ensure a successful and safe fermentation process.

e) Allow Adequate Fermentation Time: Fermentation is a time-dependent process. Different foods and recipes have varying fermentation times, ranging from a few days to several weeks. Patience is key, as the fermentation process takes time to develop the desired flavors and for the beneficial bacteria to multiply. Regularly taste your ferment to determine when it has reached the desired level of tanginess or acidity.

f) Store Fermented Foods Properly: After fermentation, store your homemade probiotic foods properly to maintain their quality and safety. Most fermented foods should be stored in a cool place, such as the refrigerator, to slow down the fermentation process and preserve their freshness. Follow specific storage guidelines provided in recipes or guidelines.

g) Be Mindful of Safety: While fermenting foods at home is generally safe, it's important to be mindful of potential risks. Use proper food safety practices, handle ingredients hygienically, and be cautious of signs of spoilage or contamination. If you have any concerns or uncertainties, consult reputable resources or seek guidance from fermentation experts.

Remember that fermentation can be a trial-and-error process, and not all batches may turn out perfectly. With practice, you'll develop your skills and preferences for fermentation techniques and flavors. Enjoy the process of creating your own probiotic-rich foods and experimenting with different flavors and combinations.

5.3 Probiotic Supplements vs. Natural Sources

When it comes to incorporating probiotics into your diet, you have the option of choosing probiotic supplements or natural food sources. Here are some considerations for both:

Probiotic Supplements:

- Convenience: Probiotic supplements offer convenience, as they come in pre-measured doses and can be easily incorporated into your daily routine.

- Specific Strains and Dosages: Probiotic supplements often contain specific strains of bacteria in measured doses, allowing you to target certain health conditions or concerns.

- Higher Concentration: Probiotic supplements can provide a higher concentration of bacteria compared to some natural food sources, ensuring a more consistent intake of beneficial bacteria.

- Shelf Stability: Probiotic supplements are typically shelf-stable and can have longer expiration dates, making them a convenient option for those who may not consume fermented foods regularly.

- Allergen Considerations: Probiotic supplements offer options for individuals with specific dietary restrictions or allergies, such as those who need dairy-free or gluten-free alternatives.

Natural Food Sources:

- Dietary Diversity: Natural food sources of probiotics provide a broader range of nutrients and dietary diversity, along with the beneficial bacteria. Incorporating a variety of fermented foods into your diet can offer additional health benefits beyond probiotics.

- Nutritional Value: Natural probiotic foods are often

nutrient-dense, providing a range of vitamins, minerals, and other beneficial compounds that contribute to overall health.

- Culinary Enjoyment: Fermented foods can add unique flavors and textures to your meals, making them an enjoyable part of your culinary experience.

- Whole Food Approach: Natural food sources of probiotics offer a whole food approach, providing a combination of beneficial bacteria, fiber, and other nutrients that work synergistically to support gut health and overall well-being.

Ultimately, the choice between probiotic supplements and natural food sources depends on your individual needs, preferences, and health goals. Some people may benefit from a combination of both, using supplements for targeted strains or therapeutic purposes and incorporating natural sources for a diverse range of beneficial bacteria and additional nutrients.

5.4 Precautions and Potential Side Effects

While probiotics are generally considered safe for most individuals, there are some precautions and potential side effects to be aware of:

a) Allergic Reactions: Some individuals may be allergic to specific strains of bacteria used in probiotic supplements or fermented foods. If you have known allergies to certain ingredients or experience allergic reactions after consuming probiotics, discontinue use and consult a healthcare professional.

b) Digestive Symptoms: In some cases, probiotics can cause mild digestive symptoms such as gas, bloating, or diarrhea. These symptoms are usually temporary and subside as your body adjusts to the introduction of probiotics. If symptoms persist or become severe, it's advisable to consult a healthcare professional.

c) Immune Compromised Individuals: Individuals with weakened immune systems, such as those undergoing chemotherapy or with severe immunodeficiency disorders, should exercise caution when considering probiotics. Consult a healthcare professional to determine the appropriateness and safety of probiotic use in these cases.

d) Pre-existing Health Conditions: If you have a pre-existing health condition or are taking medications, it's important to consult with a healthcare professional before starting probiotic supplements. They can advise on potential interactions or contraindications with your specific condition or medication.

e) Quality and Safety: When choosing probiotic supplements, opt for reputable brands that adhere to quality manufacturing practices. Look for products that contain specific strains and provide information on viable counts or colony-forming units (CFUs). Proper storage and handling of probiotic supplements are also crucial to maintain their effectiveness.

It's important to note that the effects and benefits of probiotics can vary among individuals, as everyone's microbiome is unique. If you have specific health concerns or questions about probiotics, it's recommended to consult with a healthcare professional or a registered dietitian who can provide personalized advice based on your individual needs and circumstances.